Also by Alison L. Alverson

Emotional Intelligence : 21 Effective Tips To Boost Your EQ (A Practical Guide To Mastering Emotions, Improving Social Skills & Fulfilling Relationships For A Happy And Successful Life)
Empath: An Extensive Guide for Developing Your Gift of Intuition to Thrive in Life
Empath Workbook: Discover 50 Successful Tips To Boost your Emotional, Physical And Spiritual Energy

Watch for more at www.alisonalverson.com.

Table of Contents

Empath

An Extensive Guide for Developing Your Gift of Intuition to Thrive in Life

Alison L. Alverson

Introduction

Greetings readers! Congratulations for taking the first step towards transforming your life. My understanding of what an empath is became substantial and real while I was in Mexico. I was a primary school teacher in Veracruz, for a UNICEF All-in-school initiative. This rural and rugged neighborhood was predominated by aggressive Latinos and a dislike for foreigners. The education and social system in that part of North America was quite strange for an American like me. I took great interest in the academic wellbeing of the students, often to a fault.

Maria had been absent from school for about two weeks and, as her class teacher, I was worried. Alicia struck me as a mother who was very concerned about her daughter's education. So, I went to visit the young child. Every Latino brow was raised at me, as I walked down the local neighborhood of Juarez. My presence as an American was a threat to everyone around me. It was actually a bit of irritation and a lot of anger. "TEE-chuch" Maria shouted as she ran towards me. Then Alicia joined us, and she had a very surprised look.

With barely a short conversation, she hurriedly agreed to bring her child to school the next day. The tension in her response seemed like something wasn't right and I wasn't in the right environment to question her. It seemed like she was scared that someone would find an American with her in such a neighborhood. The next day, I was in front of the blackboard teaching the students - including Maria. All of a sudden, there was a disturbing rant that caught my attention. I went out of the class to check and just at the door, Alicia walked briskly into the class with her face bruised to a pulp.

Alicia grabbed her daughter's arm and dragged her out of the class. Just before she exited, she hissed at me. I watch the two strolls down the stairs. Not long after, there was a gunshot as Alicia held her daughter closer, clueless of which direction to move on the stairs. A pickup van drove to a stop at the side of the building. Two armed men jumped out and came up the stairs. I went back into the class to check on the students, but they looked unthreatened. The bandits had been invading schools and churches frequently. Alicia ran into the class and asked me to go into hiding. Before she could explain the rationale, the Mexican bandits came into the class, "Where is the American?" At this point, there were too many questions running through my head, and I am sure you can imagine some of them. From my ironed tie to the spotless long sleeves, I was obviously the American that they were looking for. One of the armed guys pointed a gun at me with so much disgust, as if I had offended him. "Your president keeps harassing us" he said in an irate way. As he was about to shoot, Alicia jumped in front of me, knelt on the floor and started begging like her life was at stake.

How could I have begged the angry Mexican if it had not been for Alicia? She endangered her life just to protect me. She forgot the presence of her child or the other students and fought for an American. Despite the stained profile attached to Americans in that part of the Mexican city, she stood up for me. Alicia was not brave; she was not a superhero; she was only an empath. An empath is someone who can absorb other people's emotions and sometimes suffer physical symptoms due to their high sensitivity.

They develop a natural connection with absorbed emotions, and they respond appropriately. It was my experiences in Mexico with Alicia that motivated this literary expression of an empath's claim and who an empath is. The book gives an extensive overview of the characteristics and traits of empaths with Alicia as a case study. This series also addresses imaginative questions like, "What if Alicia was shot? Was her action brave?" Where should the line between been an empath and been logical be drawn? Should the line even exist? This page thriller consistently connects the inferred theories about empaths with my real-life account. At the end of this series, readers should be able to identify empaths.

This won't be that difficult as about 2 – 4% of the American population is clairsentience; a group that covers empaths. A lot of similar exercises are included in this series for a comprehensive understanding including the discussion of the causative agents of this extreme level of sensitivity. So let's dive in!

Taking this journey alone is not recommended so I highly encourage you to join our friendly community on Facebook to maximize the value you receive from this book. What often helps a lot is connecting with other like-minded empaths. People you can relate to, get support from and learn from on how to navigate this world with your unique gift. This can be an excellent support network for you.

It would be great to connect with you there,

Alison L. Alverson

To join, visit:

www.facebook.com/groups/empathsupportcommunity/

Discover Your secret Spiritual Gift

Everyone possesses a spiritual gift ...

But most people never know it

Discover and unleash your spiritual gift today ...

When you complete this short quiz

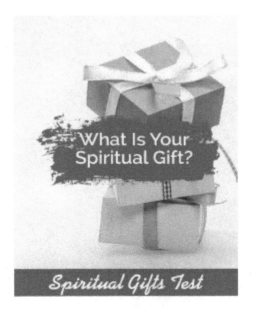

To find out your secret spiritual gift right away, visit:

https://bit.ly/3aDUiNk

Introduction to Being an Empath

Who is an empath?

An empath is a person who is deeply sensitive to the emotions and situations of those around them. This sensitivity is often to a level where they feel the emotions themselves, equipping them with the capacity to respond appropriately. Their keen interest in interacting with the emotional needs of others makes them very understanding. If the connection is deep enough, empaths can feel someone else's pains. This chapter discusses what an empath is, the traits common to an empath and how people become empaths. This connection is not restricted to humans alone as some other types of empaths interact with the needs of animals, plants, places, the environment etc.

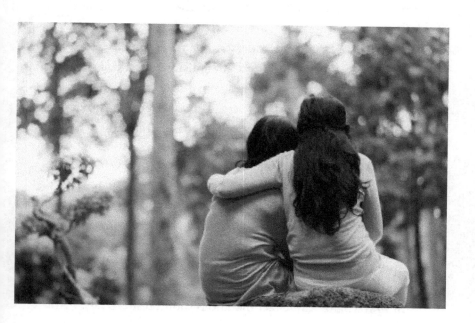

What are the traits common to empaths?

These characteristics differentiate them from Highly Sensitive People (HSP) who just have great empathy. Irrespective of the several types of empaths they all share some common traits. Here are some of the attributes common to empaths.

- **Heightened sensitivity:** This is the most common and basic trait of empaths. They tend to pick up on the feelings and thoughts of others, no matter how hidden. Empaths react and connect to these emotions like they are the subjects. This high level of sensitivity can be related to mirror neurons. Scientists theorize that these neurons read emotional cues from others and connect to their thoughts. The subtle changes in expressions, body language, and other parameters are easily noticeable by empaths. Most times these small changes are often another form of more delicate circumstances. Plant empaths can connect, understand and communicate with plants as even the most subtle organisms have things to say. The nature of plants would obviously infer that their communication is very latent. It requires extreme sensitivity to relate to the little movements of leaves and branches.

- **Overwhelming emotions:** This sensitivity can also be unintentional as it also occurs in public places. The nature of empaths leaves them vulnerable to every type of emotion. The numerous and contrasting ambiance of crowds and noisy environments can be challenging. In effect, empaths react and respond to the nature of their environments. Empaths become more effectively sensitive in quiet and serene surroundings. They internalize these feelings and respond respectively. Plant empaths often get irritated with human activities that alter or compromise the wellbeing of trees and plants. This ends up creating overwhelming emotions especially because there is very little that can be done about it. Geomantic empaths are certainly not left out. Imagine a geomantic empath that has developed a deep bond and connection with the ocean witnessing the ocean littered with plastic bottles and waste. This is common with countries that share the ocean's coastline. In some parts of Africa, the drainage and sewage system all lead into the ocean. The sight of this environmental discrimination can overly dampen the feelings and the emotions of geomantic empaths.

- **A grounded understanding of other's emotions**: One of the core traits of an empath is the ability to understand the origin of people's emotions. This understanding creates a natural connection with others. Empaths know the other party's thoughts and feelings even when they are finding it hard to express them. In such a case, empaths even help others articulate and express themselves better. An animal empath can deduce that when fleas are hovering over a dog, then a disease could be contracted. The connection they share with the animals gives them the capacity to understand and interpret every little behavior properly.

- **Useful and relevant advice**: The insights and genuine characteristics of empaths are why they are always sought after for advice and emotional support. In the course of this, empaths tend to be good listeners, willing to hear all the complex emotions. The relevant advice provided by empaths is a reflection of their understanding of other people's emotions. Emotional empaths connect with absorbed emotions but remain mentally stable enough to react appropriately or give objective and relevant solutions. Most deforesters really do not understand the negative consequence of their activities. A lot of them see deforestation as the only alternative but with the grounded understanding of an empath, relevant and resolving advice or alternatives can be offered. There is a general problem of lack of information and can be solved with relevant advice.

- **Calm and non-violent nature**: As mentioned earlier, empaths function better in a quiet and calm environment. These factors are internalized and make them easily irritated by violence. This irritation also translates into movies as they can't watch violent movies. They respond positively to calm environments and negatively to violence. It is almost impossible to find a geomantic empath that has a deep connection with disorderly and crowded places like the marketplace. This is because their subtle and sensitive nature ensures that they are only able to connect and process orderly stimuli and emotions. An Empath's vacation is most likely to be spent at the beach on a quiet day or in an isolated island. They can travel over land and watch the elephants in African game reserves. Others even spend their holidays in solitude or alone.

- **Love for pets and babies**: The pure nature of animals and babies easily appeals to the genuineness of empaths. They find it easier to appreciate and connect with pets and babies. This connection is a result of the genuineness of both parties. This is not just peculiar to animal empaths as all the types of empaths share a genuine nature and emotional purity. Hence their connection with babies and animals is natural. It is also important that the connection and likeness goes both ways.

- **Complications in relationships**: The constant closeness of empaths to someone else like a partner can be very challenging. These challenges are a result of the constant sensing of their partner's mood, irritation or feelings. The constant presence of a partner is a big drag on the empath's energy. This is even more so when the partner is very insensitive. Alicia was married to an emotionally passive man, in the person of Miguel. She takes on the burden of every emotional need. Without any form of support, she solely ensures the academic wellbeing of their daughter. Miguel discourages her nature and emotional tendencies, but she still has to care for him to maintain the required balance. Some empaths resort to staying single; others create a private room in their homes for just themselves.

● **Truthfulness:** The truthful and sensitive nature of empaths gives them the capacity to identify lies and truth. They are receptive to even the slightest social cues from others, so it is almost impossible to lie to them. This is obvious in the case of animal empaths as their nature is always true and genuine. Humans have the tendency to suppress their emotions and feelings, but empaths can always see beyond the external cues. Their developed intuitions overcome every form of emotional barrier.

● **Calming effect and emotional healing:** The connective and genuine nature of empaths makes it easy for others to open up to them. During trying times, people often seek their most empathetic friends, which is what empaths represent. The openness of others is the first step to emotional healing. The effect they have on others helps in resolving emotional baggage and unraveling unhealthy patterns. Because animal empaths understand and genuinely care, the animals tend to open up. These animals are violent to people that they cannot connect with. For example, the relationship between a dog and a dog owner becomes very affectionate over time. This is because the owner can now put meaning and interpretation to every behavioral change. The dog also gets to know the implication of every gesture of the owner. This is unlike the animal empath who gets all this connection and interaction with animals in just a moment. They do not require a very long time for the development of the connection.

● **Compassion**: Most empaths feel obligated to help people in need, without consideration of how this will come about. They place the utmost priority on helping others. They can stop every endeavor just to focus on someone else. When emotional empaths absorb the feelings of others, they don't understand everything in the instance. But they still take the risk knowing they might not be able to help. Alicia couldn't have been 100% sure that the Mexican bandit would not shoot but her compassion was hard to suppress. It is only compassion that would make plant empaths want to interact with the endangered species of plants and trees. It is safe to say that the first instinct of empaths is compassion; they go to the trouble of using their emotional energy and strength to make resolutions.

The Science of Being an Empath

The traits of empaths are closely linked with the mirror neuron system. This system in the brain enables empaths to feel the emotions of others. When empaths sense negative or sad emotions from others, the neurons in the brain become activated. The activation stimulates experiences corresponding to the ones the other person is going through. There are credible theories on empaths and how the evolution of intuition which might have resulted from biological and psychological uniqueness between empaths and others. There are several scientific theories that can explain the special attributes and behaviors of empaths.

- **Sensory Processing disorder:** This is a medical condition that makes a person struggle with processing absorbed information. The inability to properly use this input creates a magnified effect on every unit of information being absorbed. When the senses are over stimulated, they react in line with the nature of data. This can result in dizziness, anxiety or even confusion. The sensitivity is also present in the level of people's emotions. So, they are aware of the feelings of others. Some research links these traits to genetic components and others postulate that the disorder is due to abnormal brain activities. This anomaly can be in response to noise, light and other over-stimulating inputs. The disorder can also be as a result of the inability to process feelings and emotions. Alicia came to help plea for me. What if she did this because of her inability to process violence or even death? It is possible that she couldn't comprehend the situation and she acted from a faulty processing.

- **Overactive mirror neurons:** Mirror neurons are brain cells with proven connection to human compassion. These neurons are basically responsible for empathy. Empaths tend to be sad when others are hurting or happy when others are. These mirror neurons can activate reactions corresponding to those of observed emotions. In a sense, this theory tries to take the control of emotions from the empaths. The neurons are just suggestive, and this comes in a very subtle nature. An empath can still decide to be happy when others are sad or at least positive emotions can still be practiced. Nonetheless, empaths often succumb to these neurons and react accordingly.

• **Electromagnetism**: A lot of the symptoms and characteristics expressed by empaths can be explained by electromagnetism. The major question that the theory answers is if the electromagnetic field is capable of influencing the magnetic field of others. In this theory, the heart and the brain of empaths generate electromagnetic fields, which are interactive with the individual's feelings and emotions. With close emotional proximity, their energy fields interact, and information can be received, and emotions connected to. This explains the capacity of empaths to cash in on even the hidden emotions of others without deciding to. It also gives credence to the exhaustive feelings empaths suffer when in crowded and disorderly places. Their electromagnetic field interacts with so many diverse and sometimes contrasting emotions from others.

• **Hormones and chemical activities**: This theory links the level of sensitivity to hormonal levels and neuro-transmitters. The study was centered upon dopamine, a neurotransmitter that influences the human response to pleasure. The study revealed that empaths are more sensitive to dopamine than others. They require less of it to achieve pleasure. Empaths are more reactive to chemical changes in themselves and others. The little cues from the chemical changes in someone else is easily noticed and reacted to. Empaths possess a lower chemical threshold than most, so they tend to sense and react excessively. The study extensively covered dopamine but effective on most neuro-transmitters.

• **Emotion contagion**: In this theory, emotions are just contagious. A baby has a high probability of crying when there is another baby crying. People who are subject to kindness often show kindness. It is a very simplistic way of explaining the complexity of empaths. They mirror the emotions around them, internalize them, and often react more rationally. This theory puts the nature of empaths at a disadvantage because to better society, empaths need to express superior emotions and behaviors. Society wouldn't be substantially improved by empaths if empaths are just reflective of a bad society. Geomantic empaths would naturally be happy at the beach because of the nature of the emotions expressed in such an environment. The lively and vacation like atmosphere would be reflected in the empath's emotions. On the other hand, if the geomantic empath is in crowded, toxic environments the emotions are most likely going to be negative.

- **Synesthesia**: It is a medical condition that links two different traits which naturally wouldn't be connected. Individuals with synesthesia might link colors or songs. In the case of empaths, scientists believe mirror-touch synesthesia allows empaths to feel what others are feeling. In the experience, the empaths feel like the emotions are originating from them. The experiences and thoughts of the empath and the other person might not be connected but a link is derived. When Alicia saw me at gunpoint, she might have linked the scenario to a similar event in her past, which is unconnected to mine but brings out similar emotions. She connected the two experiences and effectively reacted like it was personal to her.

How does a person become an empath?

A lot of these traits were displayed by Alicia when she stuck out her neck for me. Obviously, she was driven by compassion to help an American stranger like me. She might have linked my situation to some experience in her past. She connected with it and reacted like her life was what was at stake. She also had an effective connection and communication with the bandit who surrendered to her plea. This had a calming effect on the raging Mexican who changed his mind. As an empath, she had the capacity to express my emotions appropriately while I stood in awe. Even after the men had left, she remained on the ground, wondering why she just risked her life for me. The tears might have also been as a result of her irritation towards violence. Alicia could have acted in contrast to her nature, but she would regret any consequence for the rest of her life. That emotional drag would last for a lifetime, which is incomparable to the temporary emotional drain she felt for standing up for me. There are several reasons why empaths exist in the world. The majority of these causes are temperament, genetics, trauma, and supportive parenting. **These are just psychological reasons as there are also scientific explanation for their existence and evolution:**

- **Temperament:** Some people are born with more sensitivity than others as some babies just have it when they are born. Some babies squint to the barest form of light, they cry when there are too many faces. The sensitivity of such babies evolves into the traits earlier ascribed to empaths. Geomantic empaths develop their passion and likeness for particular places and geographic sites from experiences. Their calm nature also cumulates into a natural tendency and attraction to quiet and serene places.

- **Genetics:** Some of these traits are genetically transmitted. Highly sensitive children often come from highly sensitive parents. This probability suggests the genetic influence on the traits. It is important to note that some of the traits are not inborn, they are developed. So even when empaths are born with the traits, they have to be developed or else they would end up just being empathetic. Since the traits have been related to mirror neurons, then there is a chance that is genetic.

- **Trauma**: Emotional or physical abuse can influence the extent of sensitivity of individuals. The influence is usually more extensive when the abuse is from the parents. A lot of empaths have alcoholic, depressed or narcissistic parents. This faulty parenting ironically leads to a lack of emotional defense and it creates a high level of selflessness. Their traumatic experiences are so evasive that they will always try to help others during trying times. They can easily relate other's predicaments to a traumatic event in their past. A person who lost a pet to illness or carelessness is likely to become an animal empath. There exists a natural tendency to remember the lost pet when there is a struggling pet around. This traumatic experience will ensure that the empath provides help in any way possible, because the first instinct towards animals is now compassion.

- **Supportive parenting:** These positive traits expressed by empaths can be effectively developed by good parenting. The traits and characteristics naturally evolve. Parents can direct and guide this behavioral evolution for better functioning. As earlier indicated, dysfunctional parenting can also develop this trait, but this type of empath often lacks a defined boundary. They are the ones that find it impossible to say no, even when they can't provide the solution. This is in contrast to the empaths whose traits are developed and functionally guided by the parents. They are like the trained empaths who can disconnect with absorbed emotions when necessary. Their emotional limits are established, and they observe the boundaries. Imagine having an environmentalist as a father with

19

different forms of flowers and plants around the house, in the garden and on the veranda. Such a child would naturally develop a keen interest in gardens and plants. On the other hand, a person who becomes a plant empath as a result of disasters like ground erosion as a result of bush burning and deforestation are the kind of empaths who will go the extra mile to ensure the well-being of trees and plants.

Understanding the Type of Empaths and Their Methods of Emotional Security

Types of empath

There exist several types of empaths that can be basically classified into six. Other types that have been identified but are just similar variants of these primary ones. These different classifications are as a result of the various factors and complexities associated with the traits and empathic abilities of empaths:

- **Emotional empath**: This is one of the most common classes of empaths. They have the unconscious capacity to pick up on the emotions of others. The feelings of the people around them influence the mood and feelings of emotional empaths. This type of empath is not able to differentiate their emotions from those of others. A lot of times, this kind of empath ends up being drained often due to the emotional connection.

- **Physical/emotional empath**: This type of empath can connect with the energy of others. The depth of this physical interaction makes most of the empaths end up as healers (medical doctors or into alternative medicine). During treatment, the empaths have an awareness of the patient's body and pains. They develop symptoms from other's ailments, and they can sense blockage strains in their energy fields. This type of empath that ends up as medical doctors remain unsettled until patients are cured, and problems resolved.

- **Animal empaths**: The connection with animals is predominant amongst these empaths but at a subtle level. Only a few have very deep empathy towards animals. These animal empaths devote a lot of their time to taking care of pets and animals in general. They develop the capacity to communicate and understand the expressions of animals. When a cat winks, it is trying to express the need for affection; this is one of the many interactions that are understood by animal empaths. They know when the animal is sick, they understand every behavioral change in animals and their consequences.

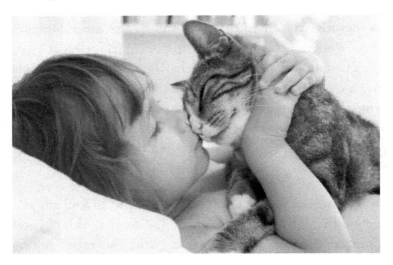

- **Geomantic empaths**: Those with this type of empathy have a sound attunement with physical landscapes or occurrences. Geomantic empaths express different emotions and moods in different environments without any apparent reason. They develop deep connections to certain places and certain things like sacred stones and certain natural figurines. A healthy love for the environment and good treatment of it ensures that geomantic empaths show a great responsibility for the wellbeing of trees and other natural objects. As earlier discussed in chapter one, empaths often get depleted and they sometimes need to recharge their energy and empathy. For geomantic empaths, they recharge from nature, the landscape, the ambiance and the serenity of their surroundings. These empaths often like to surround themselves with natural objects.

- **Plant empath**: Plant empaths are ones that have a natural passion for plants. They like to establish communication by spending time with plants. According to some plant empaths, they receive guidance from plants and trees. They are of the opinion that plants and trees have opinions, but their expressions require some level of connection and unconventional interaction. A lot of these types of empaths end up working in gardens, parks or wild landscapes where their passion is put to good use.

- **Intuitive empaths:** These empaths are subconsciously receptive to the emotions of people around. A little time with others gives them so much insight and information. They have the capacity to read the intentions behind the expression of others. It is almost impossible for them to be lied to. A lot of these empaths end up as therapists where they can construct correct opinions and profiles about patients.

Nevertheless, some empaths are a combination of various types. For instance, Alicia showed the characteristics of both an emotional and a physical empath. She didn't react according to her emotions or feelings. She keyed into my emotional energy and reacted physically like I should have. I was overwhelmed by the situation and I couldn't have reacted rationally.

Empath's precaution

The vulnerable nature of the various types of empaths requires some precautionary measures on their part. This is because they can easily be disadvantaged by their genuine and selfless nature. If the bandit had shot her, then he would have also shot me. That would have made it a double loss situation for everyone. I wouldn't assume to be the one to draw the line between empathy and reasoning but here are some of the precautionary measures. **Precautions that should be observed by empaths to avoid been drained and taken advantage of are as follows:**

- **Empath's sensitivity often draws them into others' emotions.** This can be very draining hence the need for empaths to differentiate between their emotions and those of others. There should be a line or boundary for the emotional interaction. Empaths should learn to safeguard their sensitivities. A physical empath should be able to isolate the pain of others. If they are mixed up, the reaction might not be as rational and objective as it should be. Alicia was able to isolate the emotions and feelings absorbed for me so that she made the bandit see reason. If my emotions had been mixed with hers, the plea might not have sounded like a defense for me. She might have just been begging, oblivious of the real reason for it.

- **For a lot of physical empaths, they develop health complications from being too connected and symptomatic to others' health problems.** The physical empaths need to enrich their energetic field and should undergo some form of training. Trained empaths know when to disconnect from the energy or emotions. Without training, a lot of these empaths become mentally and emotionally dampened. The truth is that this automatically reflects physically. An unhealthy state of mind will always affect one's physical health.

• **Empaths need to surround themselves with the right environment and people.** The right environment can help enrich and develop their traits. For example, geomantic empaths should acquaint themselves with the right physical landscape. Plant empaths should also stay around plants and trees to strengthen their energetic field. They should be around those they feel aligned with. Alicia stood a high chance of developing negative tendencies and addictions because of her partner. She was constantly entangled with the grievous and discriminating tendencies of her husband. She was always stressed by the emotional carelessness of Miguel, yet she felt obligated to remain helpful. Her circumstances cannot be separated from her neighborhood. A lot of the Mexicans in Juarez had the same outlook of being peasants, financially struggling yet egoistic. The biggest mistake that an empath can make is been surrounded by the wrong type of people.

• **Animal empaths spend a lot of time with animals and this interaction can easily be harmful.** A lot of studies (biological or psychological) and training can help ensure a proper and healthy relationship with animals. The compassion and the intuition that empaths live by need to be schooled. Especially for animals as a lot of diseases can be contracted from them if the necessary precautions are not taken. Training ensures that rational compassion becomes the first instinct and that the interaction observes the limits.

- **Quiet time is also an effective way for empaths to reenergize and revitalize their mental state.** Empaths do not have to do this in one place. They can take a walk, allow themselves a walk down the road or around the office. These interludes help to reposition the moods and nerves. Animal empaths typically have a lot of pets. A large part of their time is spent with animals. This necessitates some momentary time away from animals, maybe a vacation to an island or even the beach. This time spent without animals and noise helps to strengthen the emotions and improve the emotional perspective.

- **Meditation can help empaths centralize their energy.** This reduces emotional overload and ensures that empaths do not break down because of the emotions of others. In meditation, empaths are advised to escape from their active thoughts. The several minutes should be spent in complete devotion to quietness and nature. Meditation generally widens human perspective and places focus on the right path. The concept is similar to bush fallowing in agriculture where activities are halted at a farm to help it regain its value and nutrients.

How should empaths protect themselves? How should they maintain their emotional strength?

I call it a sudden twist of fate. The Mexican wanted to shoot and then he didn't. Alicia was convincing enough to save my life. After she and her daughter had left, the students stared at me, waiting for the rest of their teaching. I scrambled to the ground and told them all to go home.

The sound of their back heeled sandals tethering against the concrete floor brought back my imagination. I imagined my ribs shattering in my body supposing the trigger had been pulled. After the dust of reality had settled, I needed to thank Alicia for saving my life. I didn't want to visit them, so I poured out my appreciations in a letter. Unfortunately, the husband got to the letter first and it seemed like an affectionate letter from an admirer. He called out his wife and angrily waited for an explanation.

Alicia took the letter and tried to explain that it was from Maria's teacher in school. He asked her for my name, but she didn't respond. He then called Maria and asked for her class teacher's name. She looked at Alicia in consideration as Miguel squeezed her daughter's mouth. He forced my name out her mouth as Miguel raged and she felt there was no choice. Alicia knew he would go looking for me, so Alicia pulled all resistance to revealing my identity to protect me. She was ready for any form of violence from her husband in defending me. She compromised and complicated the relationship with her husband for a stranger. In a real sense, she was just trying to avoid violence, which was a sure outcome, now that my identity was revealed. You might ask, how should Alicia have protected herself? But the more important question is who should Alicia be protected from? Empaths are usually calm and irritated by violent tendencies. So, the relationship of Alicia to her violent husband could only be wrong or demeaning to her nature. Empaths should protect themselves by avoiding close relationships with people who have contrasting characteristics. It's easy to think that Alicia should have picked the side of her husband in my stead, but empaths naturally gravitate towards emotional victims like me. If the empathetic nature is not satisfied, they tend to isolate themselves and exist in a very conservative and depressed mood. It is important to note that Alicia wasn't just receptive to my emotions, but she also understood what the Mexican bandit was feeling. The first words of the bandit were "Where is the American?" This suggested that they had no real knowledge of who I was, and they were projecting an anger toward me. From his latter words, they were obviously angry at the international policies of the American president. The vendetta wasn't personal or that deep. Alicia probably cashed in on this line of thought. She calmed his nerves with soothing Spanish words that re-aligned his thought with the reality of not solving anything through my death. However reasonable this sounds; it came with huge risks as the Mexican could have still decided to shoot us both.

I heard intruding knocks on the door. Someone burst through the door. It was Miguel. His eyes were red. He caught my arm and then he said, "Stay far away from my wife. If I see any other letter from you, you will be in trouble!" He then took his triumphant exit. I spend the rest of that hour thinking if I had made a bad choice leaving America. Miguel's rage was not completed as he went home to Alicia. He unleashed his violence on Alicia with slaps and punches. Her empathetic nature wouldn't let her react as she ran out of the house in tears. Not long after, I heard a knock on my door again and I grabbed a plank. I pulled the door ajar and staggered out with a plank in my hand. Alicia was shocked by the sight of me as my defensive position showed vulnerability. I dropped the plank and she asked if I was okay. Personally, I believe empaths should not run from their nature. They should actually embrace their tendencies. At that point, what was most important to her was my wellbeing. With her swollen eyes she came to apologize for the actions of her husband. I was quiet for most of the time and overwhelmed by the situation. She explained everything but it seemed like he thought the American was to blame for every misunderstanding. Like Alicia, most empaths maintain or recover their strength or energy by ensuring emotional closure. She needed to talk through things with me as she felt responsible for what had happened to me. The emotional capacity of empaths can only be improved by finding this kind of closure with their feelings. Alicia would have remained worried if she hadn't talked to me. She actually left her home to balance the energy and emotions between us. In other words, they maintain their emotional strength by embracing and stretching their tendencies rather than running from them, although it is also important to observe caution and ensure that the expressed compassion is always rational. In a nutshell, empaths would only remain in a bad state of mind, when they feel responsible for some negative outcome. Above all precautions, emotional closure should be prioritized.

What Oprah Winfrey teaches us about Empathy?

The excellence and success story of Oprah Winfrey puts her in a good position to talk about empathy. She struggled through her childhood and faced a lot of difficulty in trying to become a successful black woman. There were issues with her parents and also issues in her marriage. Despite all the negative circumstances, she still remains one of the most successful women in the world. Her story is even more thrilling because she started and championed the cause of rich black women in America. In an interview, she talks about the role empathy played in getting to where she is now.

The three lessons Oprah Winfrey teaches us about empathy:

- **Empathy results from resilience in Adversity:** "The struggle of my life created empathy. I could relate to pain, being abandoned or having people not to love me." Like a lot of individuals, Oprah was a victim of abuse, assaults and serious family crisis when growing up. It took so much resilience and deliberate effort to really overcome the mental stigma that these events had on her. Now that she is renowned and accomplished, it is only natural for her to identify and want to support people going through the same. She does this with several NGOs, giveaway conversations, and even charitable organizations. Oprah teaches us that her positive application of her negative past was instrumental to the global acceptance of her brand. So we can all apply empathy to our organizational and personal life.

- **Empathy primarily fosters relationships:** "Leadership is about empathy; it is about having the ability to relate to and connect with people for the purpose of inspiring and empowering their lives." In her talk show, she uses the "rapport-talk" style where she indulges the audience in the conversations. Audience's perspective and opinions form the core of the show. Their emotions dictate the direction of the topics, this empathetic style to a TV show fosters the bond and relationship between viewers, audience and the host. Leadership or followership requires a good level of relationship and a great way to ensure a good relationship is through empathy. It puts you in a better position to understand and tolerate others.

- **Authenticity and empathy is good for personal bonding:** "Let excellence be your brand, when you are excellent you become unforgettable. Doing the right thing will always bring the right thing to you." The reason why most celebrities feel most comfortable talking on her show is because of the connection they develop with her. She is able to relate to even their most embarrassing moments and gives a platform for celebrities to properly air their views. Her unbiased and empathetic standpoints make her personal brand very authentic. The fact that she goes the extra length to help others express themselves makes her a globally renowned brand. She has been able to do this for 25 years now because she is not different from her brand. She sticks to her truth and allows people have their opinions and the global connection naturally falls into place.

The Most Struggles Empaths Prone to and Their Effects in Society

The struggles of an empath

An empath is an anomaly to a lot of persons. Sometimes their nature can even be baffling to themselves. The unique and extensive perspective can cause empaths to struggle, especially in a very complex world like the one we live in. Uncontrolled sensitivity and emotionally unhealthy relationships are some of the basic factors that can make an empath struggle. The keen interest of empaths developed towards animals, plants or even places is usually in contrast to the understanding of others. At some point, I found her behavior extreme and vulnerable.

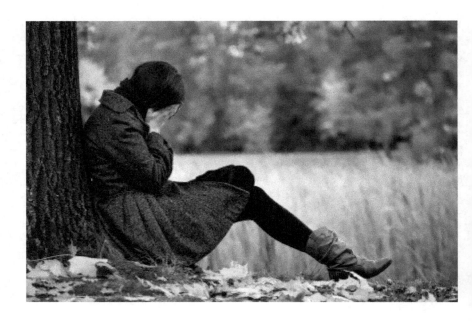

Here are some of the struggles that empaths are prone to:

● **Anxiety and depression:** These are common states that empaths find themselves in. Contrary to some opinions, it is not only as a result of their affiliation or interaction with the negative energy of others. Empaths get worried or depressed by unhealthy perceptions and negative feedbacks from others. Empaths easily attain the extreme levels of this state due to causative triggers. As earlier discussed, these triggers are the factors that make individuals become empaths. It could be temperament or unstable parenting etc. Empaths have a natural tendency to end up being anxious or depressed. Alicia was so worried about my emotional health that she left her home for a conversation with me. She needed to do this to be at peace with her nature. Environmental or plant empaths also get anxious or depressed when trees are being cut down or when plants in general are not cared for. This applies to the other types of empaths who attain this state when their peculiar passions are disregarded. Most of the time, they are handicapped when nothing that can be done about them.

● **Emotion narcissism and energy drain:** Empaths are very intuitive. They use even the most subtle emotions and social cues to determine truth or lies. This easily sounds like a great ability for empaths. But despite this ability, they are still vulnerable to people that I call emotional narcissists. They take advantage of the compassionate nature of empaths as they always want to draw empaths into their situations. Their emotional needs are usually deep and thorough, requiring so much energy from the empaths. Naturally, empaths tend to connect with these narcissists and find it difficult to retrench this emotional involvement. Untrained empaths struggle with such people a lot as they find it very difficult to disconnect. The consistent pattern of negative incidences around me made it more difficult for Alicia to associate with me. This narcissism can also be juxtaposed to an ill pet that is surely going to die. The empathetic owner knows the pet will die but will still take all the available chances to save the pet's life. With all the energy and resources expended, the pet dies and the empath remains depressed and drained.

● **Unintentional, excessive and overwhelming emotions:** Empaths often sense and receive emotions from others. This can be overwhelming in crowded environments where emotions are coming in all directions. The several emotions can be confusing and end up being mixed with theirs. With the inability to differentiate their emotions from the ones absorbed, this is obviously a struggle. This is a strong struggle because if all the emotions are taut, the connections and emotional interaction of empaths cannot be effective. This emotional struggle is also often faced by animal empaths. Some animal empaths go as far as taking in sick and homeless animals. And when the animal has recovered, they find it hard to let go of the animals. They develop a quickened connection with the animals.

● **Selflessness:** Most of an empath's focus is on others. They make every effort to resolve the emotional baggage of others. This is often done to a fault as their own emotions are neglected. After Miguel left my house, he went back home and started assaulting his wife. Alicia knew the outcome of not giving Miguel what he wanted yet she didn't. Her welfare was never the concern. She got assaulted for it and am sure when another opportunity arises, she will do the same. If that isn't selflessness, then nothing is.

- **Flexible boundaries:** Some empaths actually establish boundaries to protect themselves, but they are often not observed. Empaths generally have the inability to say "no" or disappoint others. They would rather shift the boundaries or their emotional capacity to accommodate the needs of others. Their thin and flexible boundaries leave them defenseless as they almost allow anything and everything. This encroachment has a huge probability of leaving empaths drained and irritated. But if they say no, they end up feeling guilty and depressed. It is a very confusing struggle that can only be overcome by proper training. After Alicia dragged her daughter out of the class, she hissed at me indicating a form of regret or irritation. Yet she still came back to plead for me when the bandits wanted my life. After the bandits left, she hissed like she was largely angry and irritated by the incidence. One would think she would never associate with me. But when she got bruised for holding back my identity, she still came knocking on my door. She was more concerned about my wellbeing. She seemed to create boundaries and then end up not observing them or shifting the boundaries.

The effect of empaths in society

Society can basically be divided into individualistic and communal society. An individualistic society is one in which individual achievements and accomplishments are sought after. Nobody wants to do anything for others. In the case of communal society, priority is placed on community goals and objectives. Personal accomplishments are made secondary. The effect of the various types of empaths would be discussed in relation to the direction of their influence. Do they make society more individualistic or more communal? The influence of their tendencies and traits on themselves is an important factor in evaluating their effect on society.

- *Emotional empaths have the ability to know the true emotions of others without even asking.* They see through the behaviors, reservations or any other front that people often put up to hide their emotions. This discerning ability can go a long way in rectifying tendencies like suicide and depression. A lot of suicides would be averted if only there was someone to help carry their burden and rationalize their thoughts. Nobody actually wants to die but sometimes such people just feel so depressed and worthless at that moment. These thoughts might not be true, and it would only take a mature conversation to make such people disregard the thoughts. The challenge is usually how to identify these people that have suicidal tendencies. It takes highly sensitive people like emotional empaths to discover these thoughts. Emotional empaths definitely play a very important role in the social ecosystem. Also, there are a lot of people who nurse grievous ailments without having knowledge of them.

- *Animals are a huge part of nature.* They play diverse roles in maintaining our eco-system. Unlike humans, animals' feelings are extremely difficult to understand. To help animals, the first step is identifying and understanding them. Veterinarians are usually animal empaths as they are able to connect the behavior of animals to ailments. This type of empath helps to better society by improving the wellbeing of the animals.

- *Plant empaths try to improve the society by advocating for the proper handling of plants.* Plants and trees have good influence on the environment and its ambiance. This type of empath might not really be empathic because of the benefits of the good state of the plants. A lot of them just have a natural connection with them. The effective function of a plant empath can go a long way in developing society and the ecosystem at large. More breathable air to the increased greenery are some of the benefits that comes with plants and trees.

- *Physical empaths are so connected with the pain and predicaments of others that they can feel it.* A lot of this type of empaths end up as doctors or nurses who will sometimes go out of their way to give medical care. These are the types of doctors who will go as far as helping poor patients from their own pockets. These characteristics or empathetic expressions are another form of love. With so much evil and crime, love is direly needed to create the required balance and peace in society. The other types of empaths like the geomantic and intuitive empaths also help to better society with focus on particular subjects.

The effect of society on empaths and their self esteem

The effect of society can be seen in several ways. Firstly, society realizes the important role that empaths play. In a way, there is a great emotional demand for them. Society easily takes advantage of them due to their selfless nature. Even in marriages, empaths have to carry all the emotional baggage of the family members and partners. The relevance and the demand for emotional empaths like therapists is gradually on the rise. The effect of society is different for the various types of empaths. Intuitive empaths are usually considered creepy and encroaching. Since they have intuitive knowledge of things about to happen, people consider them as weird. This is even more so when what they foretell is negative. The geomantic empath usually has implicit expressions. Their connection or irritation by geographic location and places occur internally and influence their mood but naturally does not interact with society. A lot of the geomantic empaths end up as tourists, who are constantly seeking new places that they can connect with. The serenity of the environment and the balance of nature is often offset by human activities. Some are legal and others are illegal. A lot of this balance and serenity are maintained by plants and animals. The passionate advocacy by plants and animal empaths often leave them at loggerheads with the majority of society whose activities are often unhealthy to nature in general. Society wants to be more commercial. It wants more buildings to replace the trees and the farms. Society wants animals to roam the streets un-catered for. Society shows an unhelpful dislike for some types of empaths while too much is expected from the others.

Self-esteem basically means being confident in yourself. Empaths generally struggle with confidence as a result of the absorption of other's negative emotions and the constant exposure to external energy. It is difficult to feel good about yourself when you are immersed in the energy fields of emotionally dampened people. The consistency of this emotional interaction can easily ground the self-esteem of empaths. Good self-esteem is often associated or derived from positive accomplishments and emotions. Their carriage and resolution and many emotional needs and wants leaves them very vulnerable and stressed. They are stressed about the situation of others and sometimes their inability to do anything about negative incidences or provide solutions. This results in lack of confidence and they tend to struggle with self-worth or self-esteem. When Miguel was assaulting Alicia for refusing to tell him my identity, she didn't respond or react to the violence. She simply left the house in tears. This is obviously a matured reaction and it is what a lot of empaths would do in her shoes. The point is, this kind of reaction or tendency might be as a result of lack of self-worth or self-confidence. If she really knew her worth, she wouldn't have allowed anybody to assault her without resisting it. She doesn't have to retaliate with violence but should not expect the assaults like she had deserved them.

The Uniqueness and Roles of Empaths in the Social Ecosystem

The uniqueness of empaths can only be defined with respect to others in the social ecosystem. The traits they possess don't actually start in the forms described in previous chapters. There is usually an evolution of these characteristics into empathic forms. Although the uniqueness can be glaring right from a young age, so much development and guidance goes into making a good empath.

The evolution of empath's sensitivity

Just as earlier highlighted, the evolution usually starts from birth. Some babies are just more receptive and reactive to surrounding conditions. I like to call this condition Sensory Processing Distinction. The methods of expression or out forms of their sensitivity do not remain the same as they grow. It is important to note that the direction or form of evolution is greatly influenced by parenting and upbringing in general. These traits and attributes can be guided and developed for positivity.

The first stage of the evolution is based on touch, noise and sight. At birth, the empathic ones are either hypersensitive or hyposensitive to touch. The hypersensitive ones are uncomfortable with touch and they tend to cry. The feeling of the warmth from another person's hand makes them ticklish and insecure. Most times, this tendency is cushioned by the mother as the child begins to feel comfortable with the mum's touch. Depending on the parent, the child can remain like that or the trait can be developed to a socially profitable level. Others are hyposensitive to touch; they always want to be carried around by

anyone. They tend to depend on the people around them to work or to do anything. These babies tend to cry a lot when there is nobody around.

Empaths right from a very young age are usually hypersensitive. They squint their eyes at very bright lights, they cry when they are in different environments than they are used to. They can also be uncomfortable with totally dark places as they enjoy dimly lit rooms. Parental influence is often limited as the sensitivity remains at that height through several stages of growth.

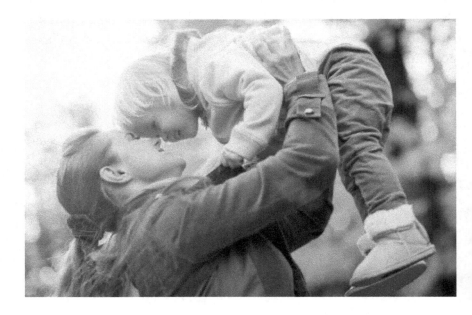

This next stage of evolution is based on allergies and behaviors. Just before the teenage years, they begin to discover the things that greatly irritate them. For some others, their parents are the ones who first cash in on their allergies and behaviors. A lot of empaths are allergic to certain types, colors or even textures of food. Sometimes it is even the smell of the food that turns them off. As a contrast they discover the smell that they are attracted to. Some children always want to go to the beach every vacation just because of the subtle smell of the ocean breeze. Some empaths don't like bathing because they hate the smell of soap. The list is exhaustive as new experiences, new allergies and passions are discovered. Empaths also exhibit sensory avoidant behaviors and sensitivity to negativity. The sensory avoidant behavior is expressed as fear of heights, easy loss of balance, fear of fast movements (ski, skating, and bicycles). They also avoid hugs and eye contact. These self-explanatory expressions are the ways in which empaths avoid their fears and insecurities. At this stage, they begin to develop sensitivity to negativity and violence. They begin to realize that they don't like violent or tragic films. They would rather stay glued to romantic and comedy films with non-violent and happy endings. At this stage, they also discover what they are good at or bad at. This next stage is based on a tripod of noise, inner-conflict and social avoidance. Most empaths are usually calm, and they get mentally energized and emotionally balanced by serene environments. They are irritated and overwhelmed by noise and loud experiences. A lot of empaths stop talking when they can't hear themselves as a result of noise. They are usually the ones that would exit the class when the noise gets too much. Empaths have a common desire for a peaceful world and existence. Their experiences are often contrasting to this desire. This results in internal turmoil or inner conflict. They struggle with their desires and the reality of how unachievable they are. At this age, empaths realize how different they are from others, but their nature won't let them challenge the status quo. As a result, they develop a tendency of social avoidance and they seek closure in personalized activities like meditation.

At the last stage, they are inevitably involved in some social activities. Some are married, others are now parents. The irritation as a result of their relationships in the social ecosystem creates difficulty in self-soothing. They have less time and less ease in calming themselves. They go through a lot of emotional roller coasters and still have to satisfy the emotional needs of their husband, wife, children and friends. At this point, a lot of outside help is needed. Close acquaintances should be able to ease the burden and create boundaries for them. The absence of this outside help can lead to suicidal tendencies and attempts. This is because they feel unfit in the world and they can't stand their incapacity in changing the narrative.

The difference between empaths and Highly Sensitive People (HSP)

Empaths and HSPs share a lot of common traits like easy emotional stimulation, quiet time, sensitivity to light and noise and distaste for crowds. HSPs are basically introverted people but empaths can be both introverts and extroverts. Empaths are typically an extension of the characteristics of HSPs. Empaths are highly receptive to the emotions, energies and physical sensations of the environment and from other people. Empaths struggle with the absorbed emotions and find it hard to distinguish theirs from those of other people. Highly Sensitive People don't typically do this. They don't get tangled with others' emotions and energies. They can sense the feelings and thoughts but do not internalize them, hence their less appropriate response compared to empaths. It is important to note that one can be both an empath and an HSP. A lot of HSPs are also empaths. Like Alicia, a lot of people can be HSP and empath at the same time. She connected with my feelings and emotions with empathy. This makes her an HSP. But a lot of the time she also got tangled with emotions and circumstances. Alicia constantly went out of her way to ensure my physical and emotional survival. The spectrum is between Narcissists, HSPs and empaths.

Empath Vs Empathy

Empathy means identifying and sympathizing with the thoughts, feelings or emotions of another person. It is a trait that all humans are capable of. Most of us can imagine ourselves in another person's shoes although empathy can both be positive and negative. With empathy, we react in correlation to the projected emotions. These characteristics are innate and can be expressed by most humans except sociopaths. It is a way of understanding other's experience from their frame of reference. In some literature, an empath is identified as someone who is empathetic. This is not totally correct because an empath is actually an extension of being empathetic. Empaths do not rely on external cues, by intuition or nature they connect with the emotions of others (even the hidden ones). Other types of empaths connect to the experiences of plants, animals etc. They do not just connect; they interact with the picked up emotions like they are theirs. Some are even symptomatic to the condition and pains of others. There are some empaths that would have to overcome their own allergies just to satisfy the emotional or physical needs of others. For example, an empath is allergic to goats and there is an infant goat that just lost his mother and the squeaking bleats indicate that the goat is lost. The emotions of the goat might rekindle a past experience of being lost. Such interaction can make the empaths take in the goat and offer to provide appropriate care. This is in spite of the allergy and shows the extent to which an empath will go to help.

Here are the key differences:

- **External trigger:** For the feeling of empathy, an external trigger or a direct cue and interaction is required. On the other hand, an empath does not require a direct interaction. Empaths can feel the emotions without even knowing the person. As explained in the several scientific theories talked about earlier, they are subconsciously receptive to all the emotions around them. Like the experiences of a geomantic empath on the beach. The feeling of the legs on the sharp sand, the ocean breeze on their skin or the sight of the moving ocean tides. The reception of these combined emotions can be overwhelming and triggering. The average empath is easily triggered because of the ability to link incidences with past

45

experiences. This is unlike an empathetic that requires direct contact (physical or emotion) before other emotions can be understood or connected to. The intuitive empaths connect experiences with emotions and are able to discern thoughts and connect with imminent incidences.

● **Healing:** Empathetic people can relate to other people's struggles and they tend to sympathize with such. Empaths connect and interact with the emotions of others so well that they can gradually walk them out of the negative emotions. They own the emotions but still maintain a healthy mental state to react, advise and respond appropriately. Their comprehensive understanding of the feelings, emotions and thoughts of others ensures their effective healing. This healing is not just emotional but can also be very physical as empaths are very caring. In truth, I felt better after the conversation with Alicia. It was easy for her to walk through the emotions while she attended to my wounds. I believe the effectiveness was from the combination of the makeup of their caring nature.

● **Accuracy of the connection:** The empath's help is even more relevant because they have the ability to determine the truth. They go in deep on the feelings, emotions and thoughts. This enables them to realize the suppressed or hidden emotions. Empath's interactions are often unintentional, so it is not influenced by unconcerned agendas. From the electromagnetic theory, even the other person can't hide the true emotions or thoughts while in the electromagnetic region of an empath. A trained animal empath can accurately discern what is wrong with a pet. This is unlike the owner who is just empathetic but does not have the ability to interpret or relate the behaviors to ailments or illnesses.

Why does the difference matter?

The differentiation of these two personalities matter because the two are actually not the same. In effect, they require different treatments and they have different motives. **Here are some of the reasons why it is necessary to differentiate between the two:**

- *A lot of empaths need training to learn how to manage their abilities without depending on them.* If the two are not differentiated and isolated from each other, empathetic people may end up getting trained for nothing. And an empath might think, training is not needed. This is important because a high percentage of empaths resort to addictions because of the overwhelming emotions. Empathy is a very good characteristic in humans and needs no form of training, but empaths need to be protected from themselves. Or at least they need to protect themselves.

- *Labeling personalities differently indicates a more detailed understanding of their different characteristics.* This gives a clearer relevance of each position in relation to others. If empaths and empathetic ones are identified and recognized under one umbrella, their different nature wouldn't be captured. If empath's tendencies are not well identified, their effectiveness will be greatly impeded. It might actually lead to self-conflict, because empaths would be considered as just any empathetic person, but it doesn't stop their tendencies. How will they feel if everyone considers them as empathetic if their sensitivity and emotional interaction is at a different level?

What empaths need to know in order to maintain their levels of empathy?

This is not about how empaths should protect themselves but how empaths can be more effective and accurate in connecting, absorbing and interacting with the emotions of others. These tips describe how empaths can harness their tendencies for emotional resolution. They also ensure that the empaths are not totally overwhelmed while being natural. **Here are some of the methods to achieve this:**

- **Grounding and earthing:** This involves connecting with the earth's energy by grounding yourself. Nature plays a major role in the lives of empaths. Contact with special earthily bodies like lying on the beach, staring at the sky at night or your foot sole in water. All this helps to tap into the energy and emotions of nature. For a lot of people, this is a way of dealing with stress but it's actually a way of laying your emotional and energy demand on nature, making the earth your source of strength and the object of your conversation. In this process, the freer, the more the connection. These techniques actually work for most empaths as their passions come from being in tune with nature. The absorbed emotions by emotional empaths have to be laid on someone or something. Fortunately, nature can accommodate a lot of this redundant energy and emotion.

- **Massage:** Massage is a way of getting out of your thoughts and emotions and placing focus on your body. This is a form of physical meditation as it puts the nerves and pores in a very relaxed state. A lot of breakthroughs have been recorded by foot massages and backrubs. It can result in having different perspectives or a different overview of how to approach the emotional demands of others. The relevance is in the distraction from your thoughts and emotions and staying in a physical pleasure.

- **Vocalization of needs and demands:** This is not to say empaths should also make others their empaths. They should just be expressive, and their personal emotions should be identified, differentiated and inputted in addressing other's emotions. This can prevent the mix of absorbed emotions and energy. Alicia continued to struggle because she was not vocal about her needs and emotions to her husband. Not that she didn't want to, but her husband seemed narcissistic. After she was done attending to my wound, it seemed like she couldn't stop talking as she had so much to say. The expression of her emotions and needs built her confidence and strength. It was actually the only time that I found her in a good mood.

- **Study and observe yourself:** Empaths need to be sensitive to themselves. If their emotions and energy are personalized enough, they are able to confine and isolate them from the emotions of others. A major stressor for empaths is the emotional mix up and acquisition of other's negative energy. Empaths should also be vocal about their feelings about their partners and friends. These feelings should not be suppressed. A lot of empaths suppress them so much that they become difficult to express or identify. Observance of oneself is the first step to personal development.

- **Practice positive emotions:** Things might not be going smoothly as the absorbed emotions can be very exhaustive. An effective way to maintain a balance is practicing positive emotions like joy, celebration or even love. This practice might not be obvious, but it can be very effective. Some of these practices include throwing an impromptu party, going on a self-date, spending time with your kids. Derive excellence and celebration-worthiness from the smallest of achievements. It might be artificial but in the long run, the positive emotions flow naturally. It is a very effective practice of overcome negative energy.

Fields where the rare gifts of empaths are relevant

The unique and special traits of empaths require certain conditions for optimum utility. The parasitic relationship often involved in by empaths extends to the workplace. As earlier highlighted, in the wrong environment (including work), the relevance of empaths can become detrimental. **Here are 14 jobs where empaths can make appropriate use of their rare gift:**

- **Nurse:** The most important part of a nurse's job is caring for patients. This is almost a perfect job for empaths as they can easily connect with patients. Their natural tendency to care for others forces patients to open up. In the case of grievous ailments, empaths can become a support system for patients. It is important to note that there is a tendency for empaths to get attached to patients and in effect act unprofessionally. For example, if a patient who the empath has developed a bond with is unable to pay the bills, she might find it difficult to let such poor patients go without treatment. Also, on busy days, the diverse accidents that are brought into hospitals can be overwhelming and irritating to such a nurse. Empaths can be a nurse in companies, private houses or hospitals.

- **Psychologists:** Psychologists basically help people with mental health issues. They study mental states, social processes and behaviors through their relationship with others and the environment. Mental health is just as serious as physical illness. According to the WHO around 20% of the world's children and adolescents have mental disorders or problems. The problems of having an unhealthy mental state is prevalent and seriously needs urgent attention and treatment. Empaths would do a great job at this because of their naturally caring, listening and understanding tendencies. Their understanding coupled with the connection with other's emotions provides them with the capacity to give proper advice. Psychologist can work in clinics, hospitals, rehabilitation facilities, health centers etc.

- **Writer:** Writing is basically a literary way of telling stories, narratives or even ideologies with words. Empaths are highly prone to powerful emotions that can lead to captivating stories and writing. This is only possible if the emotions are channeled properly. As a writer, empaths can become freelance writers, bloggers or even an author.

- **Veterinarian:** empaths are generally in tune with nature and they can communicate and interact with the emotions of the several elements in nature like animals, plants, places etc. Animal empaths have the capacity to discern the subtle gestures of animals and they understand and can relate with the animals. So empaths who are vets can easily diagnose and treat sick pets. Their interaction skills can also help with the pet owners.

- **Artist:** The experiences of empaths equip them with unique perspectives and they often conceive and express emotions in a distinct light. Art is obviously about perspective and expression; the unique and different works are often captivating and valuable. Their powerful emotions and superior energy field gives them the capacity to create unique work which can be expressed in artwork. Most of the renowned and great artworks are often influenced by negative experiences or bad emotions. Their soft spot for others and making society better increases the probability of creating relevant artwork.

- **Musician:** Similar to writers and artists, the strong emotions can be directed into good music. As a matter of fact, the music can also be therapeutic. "Confession" by Usher is one of the greatest albums of the 21st century and it was inspired by a heartbreak (negative emotions). If the emotions are put into a song, it will be highly relatable for a lot of people due to its origin.

- **Life coach:** empaths have an innate nature to help others. They get satisfied when problems are resolved. The interests of others are the priority. Being a life coach is a perfect job for empaths as they are accurately intuitive and can connect easily with emotions. Empaths are in a good position to help others achieve their goals.

- **Guidance counselor:** This is similar to a life-coach but this time, the help is provided to a child or a young adult by mentoring them. Students will be assisted to achieve academic stability and excellence. Students often fail academically as a result of a bad state of mind. Empaths can help meet the mental needs and wants of students. Also, at the age of young adults, their mindset is still malleable, and they can easily be influenced.

- **Teacher:** A teacher's job is not just academic; it also involves offering proper support and motivation. The teaching aspect might not come naturally but the latter is just as important, and empaths can execute this flawlessly.

- **Social worker:** A social worker primarily provides support for clients and individuals. This kind of job would be very suiting for empaths because of their nature and ability to influence the lives of people they get involved with. Empaths in social work should be cautious because there is a tendency to fail clients. Not all social work will have a happy ending, and this can take a deep toll on empaths. So, it is essential for an empath to develop self-care habits and the ability to withstand the inevitable disappointments.

- **NGO workers:** Non Profit Organizations are focused on particular social objectives. The nature of such organizations requires workers who are not in it for the money but for the emotional and social accomplishment. The required level of dedication and compassion needed by the social workers is easily achieved by empaths.

- **Lawyer:** Empaths can help so many lives as an attorney. It sounds like an occupation that doesn't fit an empath because of the hard mindset that people had developed of lawyers. Empaths can represent domestic violence victims, non-profit organizations or free legal counsel to charities. They should be careful not to handle more intense legal disciplines like trials. Their connection with their clients would ensure that they would go the extra mile to defend their clients.

- **Self-employed:** Self-employment is the best position for an empath to be in. They get to use their talents without stringent schedules or uncomfortable rules or even stress from the fellow workers and the work environment. Empaths can easily thrive in self-employment as they have so much control over the business. This doesn't reduce their empathetic tendency in any way, but the connection and emotional interaction will be at a comfortable pace

The Needs of an Empath

The roles empaths play in society often leave their desires unattended to. They are so involved in the lives of others that they can forget their needs or confuse theirs with the needs of others. Empathetic relationships can easily be parasitic as so much is demanded from them. This chapter discusses the needs of an empath and what they should get in return. It is obvious that Alicia wanted the academic excellence of her daughter. She also wanted to achieve this without going against the tenets of her husband. After her husband had threatened me, she needed to make sure that I was okay. From the previous chapters, it is obvious that the needs of an empath aren't particularly substantial. They basically just want to satisfy others and sometimes themselves however difficult this may be.

What do empaths want in return?

- **Emotional satisfaction:** Empaths get involved in other people's situations not just because they can't resist it but also because of the fact that they want to solve the problem. They have an addictive desire to resolve negative emotional patterns and help others out of their bad feelings. Empaths are very happy when their interactions and connection lead to breakthroughs. They might end up being stressed but the breakthroughs are another enthusiastic incentive to want to do more. I personally think that her success in preventing the bandit from killing me was a big incentive for her to stay connected or involved. She hissed and remained disgusted after the bandits left but there was a definite satisfaction.

- **A better world:** Empaths want a society where people are not emotionally or mentally stressed. They desire a world free of so much negativity. Empaths want to be part of changing the narrative and that is why they always want to help. In a better world, they wouldn't always have to carry the emotional load of people around. Environmental or geomantic empaths need the environment to be in a very good state. They want the oceans and other water bodies to be free of plastic and toxic wastes. The plant empaths need more attention to be paid to the trees and agriculture. There are some extreme plant empaths who migrate from urban areas into tents in the woods. They enjoy the ambience of cooking with firewood and the smell of the wet grasses. In general, empaths want a better and healthier society that is free from negativity. Obviously, this is almost impossibility and that fact creates a lot of pressure and stress on the empaths.

What empaths should get in return?

● **Positive feedback:** Most empaths are just as sensitive to words and opinions. They read a lot into external opinions about them. As a matter of fact, a lot of empaths won't say "no" because they don't want others to think of them as unhelpful. There is an inborn tendency to get sad when others talk badly about them. A lot of these empaths want to hear what people think about them. Positive feedback is one thing that revitalizes their empathy. I am sure when Alicia realized that her husband came to fight me, she was bothered about the opinion that I must have developed of her. She felt she was the cause of the negative event and she actually took all the blame away from her husband. In our conversation, not once did she talk ill of her husband. She was just gushing apologies and trying to make me feel better in the midst of the negativity. Her emotional satisfaction also came when she realized I wasn't angry with her but with Miguel.

- **Appreciation:** Everybody likes to be appreciated and empaths are no exception. They want people to be as sensitive to their efforts and their emotional help. This can come from their partners, friends or even children. Because of the nature of their sensitivity, the appreciation can be a small gift or a friendly outing. They strongly appreciate even the smallest form of gestures. One of the reasons why Miguel actually got angry was the unconscious joyful expression on her face while she read my letter. The appreciation seemed like what she wanted. Empaths crave appreciation and it is often because they don't get enough of it from people around them. At the end of the conversation, she really gushed about the letter.

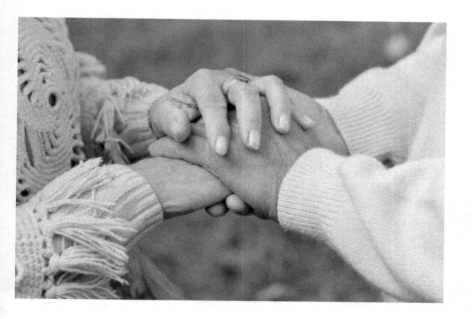

- **Better outcome:** The bad experiences of empaths in the past are easily connected to the present. Due to their highly sensitive nature, they can easily link a particular incidence with another in the past that created the same emotional effect. This creates the tendency for them to react personally to the situations of others. When Alicia heard the gunshot and the voice of the Mexican bandits coming up the stairs, she could have acted on the present emotion, which was fear. She didn't, she probably connected it with a previous incidence that provided her with fear. She might not have liked the way the past incidence ended, and she wanted to do better this time. Putting her life on the line for me might not be very rational but she didn't want to go through the negative emotions of being unable to do anything about such a situation.

Empaths and Addictions

When the absorbed emotions become too exhaustive for empaths, they often resort to mental distraction. Their heightened sensitivity gives them the capacity to hide their feelings, thoughts and emotions effectively. As a result, most people do not realize their negative state of mind. The distractions they resort to are often deep addictions. Empaths can achieve change in state of mind depending on the surrounding conditions like sound, light, noise. Picking up on the energy of everything around you (negative and positive) will naturally result in an emotional roller coaster. Addiction will always be a realistic alternative when the empaths do not have a good support system. Alicia can only take so much with the type of man she is married to. She is also a victim of the environment as the neighborhood is predominated by narcissistic Mexicans.

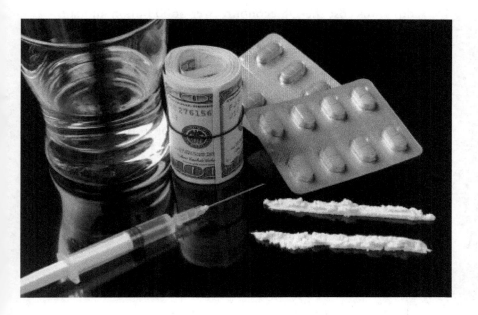

Common addictions:

- **Drugs and alcohol:** Empaths turn to drugs and alcohol to ease their empathic edginess. They drink alcohol to subdue their sensitivity and to make them less aware of the environment. The prescription sedatives, marijuana or spirits temporarily protect them from the insecurity in the world. Like every other form of addiction, it becomes counter-effective when the influence becomes latent. They remain the way they were or less. Unfortunately, some of these addictions become impossible to stop or live without at the expense of their health. According to AddictionCentre, about 20% of Americans who are depressed or have anxiety issues also have a substance abuse problem. Drug and alcohol addictions cost the US economy over $600 billion annually. These facts confirm the reality of this addiction being a viable option during depression. This easily results in apathy and social withdrawal.

- **Focus on the negative emotions:** I know a lot of empaths who seek succor in their negative emotions. They reach to their energetic fields and try to redirect and reconstruct the stressors and bad feelings. The good thing about this addiction is that it creates resistance to that particular thought or emotion. I am sure Alicia remained agitated when she wasn't sure what her husband had done to me. She wouldn't have been stable or satisfied until she had worked out her emotions with me. This suggests her focus on the negative emotion or the situation around me. It is actually this addiction that lead to emotional resolution.

- **Solitude:** In this addiction, empaths isolate themselves from everyone and everything. They ensure quality time with themselves and try to draw energy from their alternative universe. This helps them build a better perspective of their feelings and thoughts. Empaths are sometimes prone to avoiding their tendencies and focusing on themselves. I don't find this very effective as most empaths spend too much time on their negative emotions and thoughts in solitude. This is different from focusing on negative emotions as solutions are sought after. In solitude, the emotions and their resolution are avoided and cannot strengthen their mental state. Proper Solitude represents time spent alone but it actually does not mean loneliness. Statistics have it that more than 60% of lonely people are married. This suggests that a person might not be alone but yet lonely. There might be people around, but you feel lonely due to the disconnection. Solitude can help empaths know more about themselves and improve their psychological well-being.

- **Exercise:** Science has revealed a great correlation between the physical and emotions. A physical workout will help to properly channel feelings and thoughts; it also builds the mental capacity of empaths. This is like one of the most positive addictions. Exercises might take a lot of your time and get you sweating but it provides a lot of mental stamina and stress relief as a consequence. Exercises generally increase the heart rate, which eventually results in greater emotional strength. The truth is that exercise is a solution to a lot of disorders and negative conditions.

- **Herbs:** Some empaths seek to manage their anxiety and emotional depression with native herbs rather than a doctor's prescription. The use of alternative medicine in combatting emotional issues is gradually growing globally. It is important to note that a lot of the herbs do not have scientific backing. Proper regulations are not provided for these herbs unlike foods and drugs. Some of the widely used herbs used by empaths globally include St. John's wort, Ginseng, Chamomile, and Lavender etc. In a nutshell, herbal supplements are not an adequate substitute for traditional medicine. The herbs have a potential to cause serious side effects, they can also interact with other drugs due to their chemical make-up. To be on the safe side, empaths should consult a doctor before ingestion of any kind of drugs or herbs.

- **Food:** Empaths can raise their vibrations by ingesting organic foods. These highly vibrational foods can help boost the mood and their strength. The strength is required to overcome the emotional highs and lows. A large body of proof (although not direct evidence) now shows the correlation between food and mental health. A healthy diet can be very influential on the state of mind. Unfortunately, empaths often indulge in unhealthy diets while experiencing anxiety or when they are in a negative state of mind. Some empaths focus on junk food and just try to distract themselves, but this is very unhealthy both physically and mentally.

- **Sexual activities:** For a lot of people, orgasm is a heightened way of calming down. They distract themselves with the pleasure of their sexual desires. Some masturbate while others indulge in even more extreme sexual activities. This is one of the addictions that often make the feelings and self-thought worse than before, when it is done wrong or against one's beliefs. Nonetheless, there are several physical and mental benefits associated with orgasm. A spiritual empath can often feel less self-worth after immoral sexual activities like masturbation and fornication.

- **Gambling:** The unpredictability and the high stakes involved in gambling can easily get empaths engrossed. The possibility of a loss, the thrill of winning can temporarily cover the negative emotions and stressors. This is a very unhealthy addiction as empaths can also end up losing a lot thereby making their mental state worse than they were.

How empaths should deal with addictions

These addictions can be very hard to deal with especially by empaths. This is because of the consistent emotional roller coaster that they tend to experience. The lack of a good support system can also increase the tendency of addiction. Due to the numerous forms of addiction, empaths are likely to find a particular addiction that is effectively magnetic to them. Addictions are usually non-economical and irrational, which is why they shouldn't be held on to. **There are some action steps that can be used to deal with the addictions:**

- *Identify your addictions*: The first step is to identify your addictions. There should be an evaluation of the addictions, questions should be raised and answered. How often is the addiction? Should you turn to another form of addiction or not? This identification will only be effective if the empath needs to be compassionate and easy with themselves. Self-denial is very prevalent amongst empaths, as they are scared of the way the world will perceive them if everyone knows about their addiction. Until the addictions are identified, recognized and owned, the solution is not easy. For example, Alicia had an addiction of focusing on negative emotions. She remained unsettled until she was sure the intuitions and emotions were balanced and positively executed. If Alicia did not know about this addiction, it couldn't be resolved. For her, she may just see it as her own caring nature

● *Secondly, empaths need to realize that no external factor can overcome their addictions.* The refuge or solution can only be evoked from the inside. Empaths just have to accept their tendencies and know how to control the emotions and energy. This is to ensure that they are not overwhelmed and do not resort to addiction. Empaths need to dig in deep to develop closure and handle their feelings. They can get succor from their support systems or professional psychologists. Even then, nothing can be achieved without empaths playing their part in self-worth and self-comfort. The process of overcoming addictions can be lifelong.

● *Thirdly, empaths can indulge in psychotherapy; this is a very professional and effective way of addressing addictions.* It is a diverse range of treatments that can resolve mental health issues, negative emotions or even disorders. It can help empaths understand themselves and ensures dominance of the positive emotions. Psychotherapy often yields a lot of breakthroughs in depression, self-esteem and addictions. In psychotherapy, priority is placed on conversations and not medication. This is why it is often called "talking treatment." It is a two-way treatment and it often requires a good relationship between the client and the therapist that is built on trust. Psychotherapy comes in different forms and through different means for an amount of time dependent on the depth of the illness or disorder.

Conclusion

Empaths possess a very complex and delicate nature; this provides them with emotional capacity to care for others. All the various types have important roles to play in society often at the expense of their mental and physical health. This puts utmost priority on the observance of precautions and emotional boundaries. Empaths should surround themselves with like minds that can offer support when their negative tendencies are becoming difficult. The absence of these defeats every form of training that can be obtained. If Alicia had a very sensitive husband, she would have found it much easier to cope with the negative emotions. Her genuine nature always prompted the Mexican wife to her first intuition, which was compassion. Alicia would always connect or try to help people whose emotions she could relate to. I had to dissociate myself from her so that she didn't get hurt while trying to help me. This uncontrollable tendency expressed by empaths requires training to ensure mental and emotional safety. The traits of empaths evolve, and they need to be guided and developed. Parents have a huge role to play in how their personality turns out. Empaths play a very important role in our society and they should be encouraged and appreciated. This also puts an obligation on non empaths to respect the boundaries of empaths and not overwhelm them with negative energy. Empaths often have the inability to say no and will take so many risks to help others. In the light of these emotions, they develop bad tendencies and addictions. A lot of empaths also resort to suicide when there is no proper support system. Some of these tendencies can be easily be averted with conversation. **Here are some of the symptoms of suicidal tendencies:**

- Sadness and feeling of worthlessness

- Frustration and irritability

- Easy loss of interest

- Over sleeping

- Fatigue

- Concentration problem

- Changes in appetite

A lot of the time, some of these attributes can be suppressed but a combination of these often shows suicidal tendencies. The onus is on us all, both empaths and non-empaths to be sensitive to each other. Just a conversation can save a person's life.

Being an empath is a gift to this world which is full of egoism, greed, fear and massive pain and your sensitivity is an immense blessing. Imagine what world would be like if we were all sensitive and caring for each other.

Taking this journey alone is not recommended so I highly encourage you to join our friendly community on Facebook to maximize the value you receive from this book. What often helps a lot is connecting with other like-minded empaths. People you can relate to, get support from and learn from on how to navigate this world with your unique gift. This can be an excellent support network for you.

It would be great to connect with you there,

Alison L. Alverson

To join, visit:

www.facebook.com/groups/empathsupportcommunity/

Finally, thank you again for grabbing my book! Your opinion matters! Please share your thoughts about my book on the platform you bought from and don't be shy, the more information, the better. Click here: : https://books2read.com/u/4Ek1Qg

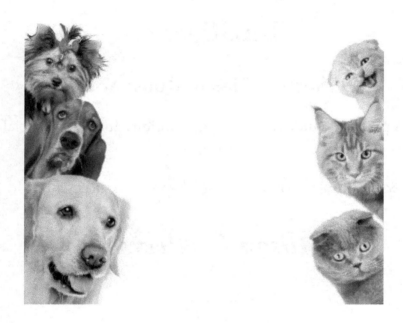

Thank you and good luck!

A Bonus Chapter Of My Book:

Emotional

Intelligence

21 Effective Tips to Boost Your EQ

A practical guide to mastering emotions, improving social skills

& fulfilling relationships for a happy and successful Life

Alison L. Alverson

The trademarks that are used are without any consent, and the publication of the trademark is without permission or backing by the trademark owner. All trademarks and brands within this book are for clarifying purposes only and are owned by the owners themselves, not affiliated with this document

What are Emotions?

Emotions are feelings that come into your mind and that affect how you react to given stimuli. You feel joy when you think of certain things, or you feel disgust at things that fall outside the scope of the acceptable. These are normal reactions that your brain uses to balance your reactions to the things that happen around you. Thus, sadness and all of the emotions you feel are affected by outside influence. They can also be triggered by your reactions to outside influence, so you can't blame the world entirely for the way that you feel. You can, however, blame your reaction to those circumstances and that's something that you have control over. You may not know it yet, but we all do, and emotional intelligence is what makes the difference. Those who do not have emotional intelligence may find themselves experiencing the negativity of emotions such as:

- Anger

- Frustration

- Jealousy

- Rage

But these are not the only negative emotions. Negative emotions are those, which cause a negative reaction within your mind. You may say that you have no control over these, but when you adopt an emotionally intelligent stance, you will find that you have more control than you give yourself credit for because your approach is different. Let's look at the seven basic emotions:

- **Anger**

71

- **Happiness**

- **Sadness**

- **Fear**

- **Surprise**

- **Contempt**

- **Disgust**

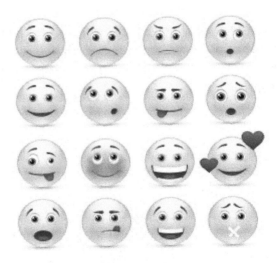

If you look at that list, you will see that more of them are negative than positive and it may surprise you to find that the mind thinks negative thoughts more than it thinks positive ones. So what's going on in the mind when it becomes emotional? Well, you would have to look for scientific proof of what's going on, but to you, you feel overwhelmed by the negativity or can even feel euphoric when you experience the joy of happiness. Why would these different emotions have such a profound effect on the way that you relate to your life? These were all questions that I had about emotions when I was taking the same journey as you are and my findings were rather enlightening.

According to neuroscientist Antonio Damasio, the feelings that we get as humans derive from external influences and he has done much work to try and determine what happens when an emotion is evoked. Damasio explains that we associate feelings with emotions and assume that certain things will happen following experiencing something that evokes a certain emotion. What's actually happening inside the brain is that certain reactions to a stimuli are triggered because the body is going into a response to what we have seen. Thus, it's common that we feel our heartbeat increasing when we are stressed. We may find that blood pressure rises or that we have sweaty palms. That's when we experience feelings such as pain.

So how do we gain better control of the way that external influences make the body react? You have to turn to science to find the answers to that. PET scanning and MRI studies show that different areas of the brain are affected by different emotions and that means that once we know the reactions, we can alter our emotions to help ourselves to remain calm and subjective, rather than simply going with the emotion being felt. Let's take a look at the way the emotion of happiness sparks off activity in different areas of the brain.

Happiness – This affects the right frontal cortex. There are also feelings within the amygdala or center for feelings and the awareness part of the brain in the frontal cortex.

There are a whole load of references which show you the different areas of the brain affected by emotions, but more interesting than that is the work that is being done by the scientific world and the Dalai Lama based upon MRI scans that were done on Buddhist monks. These experiments were done at the New York University and showed that monks were able to control the see-sawing effect of the brain jumping from one emotion to the next or from outside influence to internal influence. Dr. Josipovic, Research Assistant and Adjunct Professor at the New York University stated:

"Meditation research, particularly in the last 10 years or so, has shown to be very promising because it points to an ability of the brain to change and optimize in a way we didn't know previously was possible."

If you need further proof of this link, then watching a video by a neuroscientist may awaken you to the truth about the way that the brain reacts to the world around you and backs up the claims that people who experience compassion and humility in their approach to life tend to find that their emotions are more balanced and easier to live with. Dr. Sarah Lazar makes interesting points based on her experience as a neurosurgeon and upon her own trial at controlling emotions with the use of meditation. In her case, the results were quite amazing, particularly since she was not expecting the results that she got. She found that meditational practice could actually change the shape of part of the brain and that this change brought about peaceful thoughts and the ability to be more compassionate and capable of using emotions to positive effect.

The process of thinking in an emotional way and what it does to the brain

You may think that emotions are just thoughts, but they trigger off certain actions in the brain. For example, an MIT study revealed how there are two areas in the brain that process emotions – these are located within the amygdala area of the brain. Knowing this, experiments were done on mice to watch the activity within the brain during instances when the mice were offered pleasurable reward in the way of sugar cubes. It was certainly proven that negative effects and positive effects caused different reactions in the brain and that the amygdala area of the brain connects to different regions, which are triggered into action by the thought of reward or by negativity. What the scientists said after this experiment was:

"We are exploring the interactions between these different projections, and we think that could be a key to how we so quickly select an appropriate action when we're presented with a stimulus,"

This is also backed up by the idea that the habits that we adopt will also affect the emotional response of the human being to different stimuli. Thus, for one person a very positive stimuli could prove negative to someone else. Therefore, you have to know your own habits and the emotions that are triggered by certain actions within your life before you can control those reactions. Look at the sense of reward, for example. If an emotion leads you to some kind of reward, then you feel good about it. However, if it doesn't, it can lead to negative thoughts and negative consequences. It is important therefore that you note down the feelings or emotions that you experience during the course of a day and watch for differences in your comportment or attitude as these will have been events that are triggered within the amygdala region. In the case of the meditators, these were people who were able to balance the effects and therefore did not feel extreme emotions and were able to feel the bliss of happiness.

How emotions influence our thinking

If you experience a negative emotion, you are likely to analyze it and thus make it larger than it originally was. People who are depressed tend to over analyze and are unable to see any reward at the end of their thinking. However, people who are well balanced and whose lives are considered to be within "norms" can still over-react to a stimuli. As I said in the opening, I got mad at the man crossing the street. In my case, the shock of what was happening that was beyond my control triggered anger, but if you allow outside influences to do that to you, then you are not fully in control of the life that you are living. In fact, you are doing exactly what Warren Buffett suggests and letting people control your life and your response to life. It's like letting go of responsibility and making everyone around you to blame for the way that you feel. In fact, you are the person in the driving seat if you wish to be, and that's the purpose of this book, to bring you to a place where you actually are.

If you have self-esteem problems, these also come from an outside influence in many cases. For example, how many times have people told you that you are inadequate in some way? Your parents may have derided you for your choices. Your friends may not like your sense of style. You may be overweight and measure yourself against society norms, but the point of it all is that it's the way that you see it that matters and if you can adjust your own view of self, you can get over the fact that emotions are now in turmoil and take back control of your own life. The first fact to face is that whatever emotions are doing to you, as an individual, your thoughts and actions are being influenced by them. Thus, the less you expose yourself to negative influences or allow them to become negative, the more likely you are to feel in control of your emotions. It is a case of being in control of the way that you react to any given stimuli. Yes, of course, you will be sad sometimes, but that doesn't have to affect your thought processes if you know how to handle sadness. The best thing about emotional intelligence is that you get to drive the car and that's when life gets really interesting.

Emotions can trigger a spiral of negative thoughts or euphoria to the extreme. However, when you know more about how it all works and are able to harness this power, you find that you are more receptive to the emotions being felt by others and that you are totally in control of your own emotions and they do not trigger so much negativity that you become out of control. Your inner strength will ensure that even when you are met by negative emotions, you will have the ability to cope with them in an emotionally intelligent manner. Think about the last time that you encountered a negative emotion. Someone said something that made you angry. The situation is that you can either judge this as being a passing event or you can do what most people do and blow it up into a huge problem that is larger than life. Most people do the latter, just like I did when someone crossed the road in front of me. By the time you have finished reading this book, you will know how to better deal with the thought processes that follow your emotions, but you will also know how to control those emotions in the first place, by introducing a different set of standards – those that do not judge.

Discover Your secret Spiritual Gift

Everyone possesses a spiritual gift.....

But most people never know it.

Discover and unleash your spiritual gift today ...

When you complete this short quiz

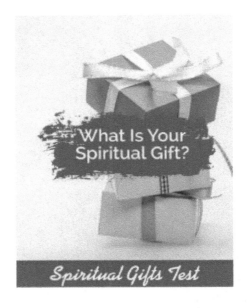

To find out your secret spiritual gift right away, visit: https://bit.ly/3aDUiNk

GOOD LUCK

Don't miss out!

Visit the website below and you can sign up to receive emails whenever Alison L. Alverson publishes a new book. There's no charge and no obligation.

https://books2read.com/r/B-A-RQLJ-EYCFB

BOOKS 2 READ

Connecting independent readers to independent writers.

Did you love *Empath: An Extensive Guide for Developing Your Gift of Intuition to Thrive in Life*? Then you should read *Empath Workbook: Discover 50 Successful Tips To Boost your Emotional, Physical And Spiritual Energy* by Alison L. Alverson!

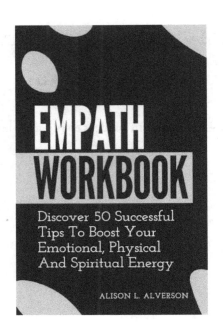

Stop hiding your empathic gifts....

Are you **constantly suffering** from adrenal fatigue, mood swings, being overwhelmed and drained in crowds?

Would you like to be able to increase your ability and control your emotional and spiritual energy?

Want to start living as your true self but don't know where to begin?

Being an Empath is a beautiful blessing, but it can also physically affect your body as well as mentally. Often, empaths can be **overwhelmed** with love and fear and find the whole process exhausting.

In EMPATH WORKBOOK, you'll discover **50** tips for understanding your energy packed with effective exercises, journal prompts, and tools like reiki, smudging, crystals, and oracle cards which will catapult you right on the path of self-discovery and self-acceptance.

In *EMPATH WORKBOOK*, you will unlock practical skills and tactics such as:

How to set **healthy boundaries** and maintain a **healthy diet**The key to understanding **Kundalini energy**Meditation techniques and **chakra healing**Secrets to help empaths maintain their closest relationshipsThe most14 useful tools every empath should masterHow to overcome common problems like **insomnia** and **psychic attacks**How to maintain your physical and mental healthHow to embrace your **shadow self**How to control your emotionshow to avoid and heal **energy cords and hooks**How to discharge and transform **negative energy**The **secret tip** empaths should know about to live happilyThe powerful empathy technique you never heard aboutThe great influence of **aura, Cymatics** and **binaural beats** on empathsThe three amazing **essential oils** for empaths to feel groundedAnd much, much more

EMPATH WORKBOOK is the ultimate navigational guide to awakening, understanding, and controlling your energy to be happy, healthy, and true to yourself.

Step out of the shadows and let this book teach you how to shine unapologetically bright as who you truly are.

Buy it now

Read more at www.alisonalverson.com.

Also by Alison L. Alverson

Emotional Intelligence : 21 Effective Tips To Boost Your EQ (A Practical Guide To Mastering Emotions, Improving Social Skills & Fulfilling Relationships For A Happy And Successful Life)
Empath: An Extensive Guide for Developing Your Gift of Intuition to Thrive in Life
Empath Workbook: Discover 50 Successful Tips To Boost your Emotional, Physical And Spiritual Energy

Watch for more at www.alisonalverson.com.

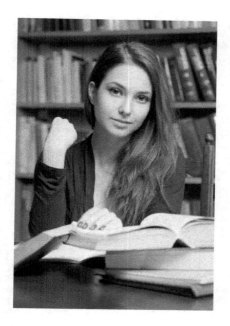

About the Author

Alison L. Alverson is an American and accomplished self-published author. She is an empath, who has spent nearly one decade, since awakening, mastering her empathic nature. She studied various psychological techniques and attended spiritual healing workshops from a variety of traditions.

She has a burning passion and an open spirit to help empaths, who are the healers, the nurturers, and the highly sensitive persons, manage their empathy without getting drained and teach them strategies to thrive as an empath by sharing with them her experiences and practical tips that helped her. She wants to grow continuously, and she wants to encourage empaths to do the same through taking consistent actions.

Alison loves to travel and finds her passion in writing books. She is a social person and loves sitting with people and listening to them. In her free time, she likes taking photos, especially outdoors, and listening to the sound of nature. Alison loves to hear from her dear readers.

Feel free to email her at alisonalverson12@gmail.com

Read more at www.alisonalverson.com.